SOUTH BEACH COOKBOOK

MAIN COURSE - 60+ Breakfast, Lunch, Dinner and Dessert Recipes for a healthy weight loss

TABLE OF CONTENTS

BREAKFAST 7
BLUEBERRY PANCAKES 7
BLACKCURRANT PANCAKES 9
CANTALOUPE PANCAKES 11
COCONUT PANCAKES 12
CHERRIES PANCAKES 13
MANGO MUFFINS 14
NECTARINE MUFFINS 16
PAPAYA MUFFINS 18
PLANTAIN MUFFINS 20
PLUMS MUFFINS 22
PRUNES MUFFINS 24
CHEESE OMELETTE 26
PARSLEY OMELETTE 28
ONION OMELETTE 30
BEETROOT OMELETTE 32
BELL PEPPER OMELETTE 34
CUCUMBER GUACAMOLE BITES 36
GREEK YOGURT AND TAHINI DIP 37
HAM AND DILL BITES 38
ROASTED ASPARAGUS IN HAM 39
LUNCH 41
SPINACH FRITATTA 41
TURNIP FRITATTA 43
SQUASH FRITATTA 45

HAM FRITATTA	47
ONION FRITATTA	49
FRIED CHICKEN WITH ALMONDS	51
FILET MIGNON WITH TOMATO SAUCE	53
ZUCCHINI NOODLES	55
GREEN BEANS WITH TOMATOES	56
ROASTED CAULIFLOWER RICE	57
CAPRESE SALAD	58
BUTTERNUT SQUASH SALAD	59
TURKEY SALAD	60
SHRIMP SALAD	61
CANTALOUPE SALAD	62
CORN SALAD	63
SALMON EGG SALAD	64
QUINOA SALAD	65
GREEK SALAD	66
AVOCADO SALAD	67
DINNER	69
SIMPLE PIZZA RECIPE	69
ZUCCHINI PIZZA	71
CAULIFLOWER RECIPE	72
BROCCOLI RECIPE	73
TOMATOES & HAM PIZZA	74
ROASTED JALAPENO SOUP	76
PARSNIP SOUP	78
SPINACH SOUP	80

CUCUMBER SOUP 82

SWEETCORN SOUP 84

SMOOTHIES 87

GREEN SMOOTHIE 87

WAKE UP SMOOTHIE 88

RASPBERRY SMOOTHIE 89

CHOCOLATE SMOOTHIE 90

PROTEIN SMOOTHIE 91

SUNSHINE SMOOTHIE 92

MANGO SMOOTHIE 93

PEACH SMOOTHIE 94

PUMPKIN SMOOTHIE 95

Copyright 2019 by Noah Jerris - All rights reserved.

This document is geared towards providing exact and reliable information in regards to the topic and issue covered. The publication is sold with the idea that the publisher is not required to render accounting, officially permitted, or otherwise, qualified services. If advice is necessary, legal or professional, a practiced individual in the profession should be ordered.

- From a Declaration of Principles which was accepted and approved equally by a Committee of the American Bar Association and a Committee of Publishers and Associations.

In no way is it legal to reproduce, duplicate, or transmit any part of this document in either electronic means or in printed format. Recording of this publication is strictly prohibited and any storage of this document is not allowed unless with written permission from the publisher. All rights reserved.

The information provided herein is stated to be truthful and consistent, in that any liability, in terms of inattention or otherwise, by any usage or abuse of any policies, processes, or directions contained within is the solitary and utter responsibility of the recipient reader. Under no circumstances will any legal responsibility or blame be held against the publisher for any reparation, damages, or monetary loss due to the information herein, either directly or indirectly.

Respective authors own all copyrights not held by the publisher.

The information herein is offered for informational

purposes solely, and is universal as so. The presentation of the information is without contract or any type of guarantee assurance.

The trademarks that are used are without any consent, and the publication of the trademark is without permission or backing by the trademark owner. All trademarks and brands within this book are for clarifying purposes only and are the owned by the owners themselves, not affiliated with this document.

Introduction

South Beach recipes for personal enjoyment but also for family enjoyment. You will love them for sure for how easy it is to prepare them.

BREAKFAST

BLUEBERRY PANCAKES

Serves: **4**

Prep Time: **10** Minutes

Cook Time: **20** Minutes

Total Time: **30** Minutes

INGREDIENTS

- 1 cup whole wheat flour
- ¼ tsp baking soda
- ¼ tsp baking powder
- 1 cup blueberries
- 2 eggs
- 1 cup milk

DIRECTIONS

1. In a bowl combine all ingredients together and mix well
2. In a skillet heat olive oil

3. Pour ¼ of the batter and cook each pancake for 1-2 minutes per side
4. When ready remove from heat and serve

BLACKCURRANT PANCAKES

Serves: **4**
Prep Time: **10** Minutes
Cook Time: **30** Minutes
Total Time: **40** Minutes

INGREDIENTS

- 1 cup whole wheat flour
- ¼ tsp baking soda
- ¼ tsp baking powder
- 1 cup almonds
- 2 eggs
- 1 cup milk
- 1 cup blackcurrant

DIRECTIONS

1. In a bowl combine all ingredients together and mix well
2. In a skillet heat olive oil
3. Pour ¼ of the batter and cook each pancake for 1-2 minutes per side

4. When ready remove from heat and serve

CANTALOUPE PANCAKES

Serves: **4**

Prep Time: **10** Minutes

Cook Time: **20** Minutes

Total Time: **30** Minutes

INGREDIENTS

- 1 cup whole wheat flour
- ¼ tsp baking soda
- ¼ tsp baking powder
- 2 eggs
- 1 cup milk
- 1 cup cantaloupe

DIRECTIONS

1. In a bowl combine all ingredients together and mix well
2. In a skillet heat olive oil
3. Pour ¼ of the batter and cook each pancake for 1-2 minutes per side
4. When ready remove from heat and serve

COCONUT PANCAKES

Serves: **4**
Prep Time: **10** Minutes
Cook Time: **20** Minutes
Total Time: **30** Minutes

INGREDIENTS

- 1 cup whole wheat flour
- ¼ tsp baking soda
- ¼ tsp baking powder
- 1 cup coconut flalkes
- 2 eggs
- 1 cup milk

DIRECTIONS

1. In a bowl combine all ingredients together and mix well
2. In a skillet heat olive oil
3. Pour ¼ of the batter and cook each pancake for 1-2 minutes per side
4. When ready remove from heat and serve

CHERRIES PANCAKES

Serves: **4**

Prep Time: **10** Minutes

Cook Time: **30** Minutes

Total Time: **40** Minutes

INGREDIENTS

- **1 cup whole wheat flour**
- **¼ tsp baking soda**
- **¼ tsp baking powder**
- **2 eggs**
- **1 cup milk**
- **1 cup cherries**

DIRECTIONS

1. In a bowl combine all ingredients together and mix well
2. In a skillet heat olive oil
3. Pour ¼ of the batter and cook each pancake for 1-2 minutes per side
4. When ready remove from heat and serve

MANGO MUFFINS

Serves: **8-12**

Prep Time: **10** Minutes

Cook Time: **20** Minutes

Total Time: **30** Minutes

INGREDIENTS

- 2 eggs
- 1 tablespoon olive oil
- 1 cup milk
- 2 cups whole wheat flour
- 1 tsp baking soda
- ¼ tsp baking soda
- 1 tsp ginger
- 1 tsp cinnamon
- 1 cup mango

DIRECTIONS

1. In a bowl combine all dry ingredients
2. In another bowl combine all dry ingredients

3. Combine wet and dry ingredients together
4. Pour mixture into 8-12 prepared muffin cups, fill 2/3 of the cups
5. Bake for 18-20 minutes at 375 F
6. When ready remove from the oven and serve

NECTARINE MUFFINS

Serves: **8-12**
Prep Time: **10** Minutes
Cook Time: **20** Minutes
Total Time: **30** Minutes

INGREDIENTS

- 2 eggs
- 1 tablespoon olive oil
- 1 cup milk
- 2 cups whole wheat flour
- 1 tsp baking soda
- ¼ tsp baking soda
- 1 tsp cinnamon
- 1 cup nectarine

DIRECTIONS

1. In a bowl combine all dry ingredients
2. In another bowl combine all dry ingredients
3. Combine wet and dry ingredients together

4. Pour mixture into 8-12 prepared muffin cups, fill 2/3 of the cups
5. Bake for 18-20 minutes at 375 F
6. When ready remove from the oven and serve

PAPAYA MUFFINS

Serves: **8-12**

Prep Time: **10** Minutes

Cook Time: **20** Minutes

Total Time: **30** Minutes

INGREDIENTS

- 2 eggs
- 1 tablespoon olive oil
- 1 cup milk
- 2 cups whole wheat flour
- 1 tsp baking soda
- ¼ tsp baking soda
- 1 tsp cinnamon
- 1 cup papaya

DIRECTIONS

1. In a bowl combine all dry ingredients
2. In another bowl combine all dry ingredients
3. Combine wet and dry ingredients together

4. Pour mixture into 8-12 prepared muffin cups, fill 2/3 of the cups
5. Bake for 18-20 minutes at 375 F
6. When ready remove from the oven and serve

PLANTAIN MUFFINS

Serves: **8-12**

Prep Time: **10** Minutes

Cook Time: **20** Minutes

Total Time: **30** Minutes

INGREDIENTS

- 2 eggs
- 1 tablespoon olive oil
- 1 cup milk
- 2 cups whole wheat flour
- 1 tsp baking soda
- ¼ tsp baking soda
- 1 tsp cinnamon
- 1 cup plantain

DIRECTIONS

1. In a bowl combine all dry ingredients
2. In another bowl combine all dry ingredients
3. Combine wet and dry ingredients together

4. Pour mixture into 8-12 prepared muffin cups, fill 2/3 of the cups
5. Bake for 18-20 minutes at 375 F
6. When ready remove from the oven and serve

PLUMS MUFFINS

Serves: **8-12**
Prep Time: **10** Minutes
Cook Time: **20** Minutes
Total Time: **30** Minutes

INGREDIENTS

- 2 eggs
- 1 tablespoon olive oil
- 1 cup milk
- 2 cups whole wheat flour
- 1 tsp baking soda
- ¼ tsp baking soda
- 1 tsp cinnamon
- 1 cup plums

DIRECTIONS

1. In a bowl combine all dry ingredients
2. In another bowl combine all dry ingredients
3. Combine wet and dry ingredients together

4. Pour mixture into 8-12 prepared muffin cups, fill 2/3 of the cups
5. Bake for 18-20 minutes at 375 F
6. When ready remove from the oven and serve

PRUNES MUFFINS

Serves: **8-12**

Prep Time: **10** Minutes

Cook Time: **20** Minutes

Total Time: **30** Minutes

INGREDIENTS

- 2 eggs
- 1 tablespoon olive oil
- 1 cup milk
- 2 cups whole wheat flour
- 1 tsp baking soda
- ¼ tsp baking soda
- 1 cup prunes

DIRECTIONS

1. In a bowl combine all dry ingredients
2. In another bowl combine all dry ingredients
3. Combine wet and dry ingredients together

4. Pour mixture into 8-12 prepared muffin cups, fill 2/3 of the cups
5. Bake for 18-20 minutes at 375 F
6. When ready remove from the oven and serve

CHEESE OMELETTE

Serves: **1**
Prep Time: **5** Minutes

Cook Time: **10** Minutes

Total Time: **15** Minutes

INGREDIENTS

- 2 eggs
- ¼ tsp salt
- ¼ tsp black pepper
- 1 tablespoon olive oil
- ¼ cup cheese
- 1 cup cheese
- ¼ tsp basil

DIRECTIONS

1. In a bowl combine all ingredients together and mix well
2. In a skillet heat olive oil and pour the egg mixture
3. Cook for 1-2 minutes per side

4. When ready remove omelette from the skillet and serve

PARSLEY OMELETTE

Serves: **1**
Prep Time: **5** Minutes
Cook Time: **10** Minutes
Total Time: **15** Minutes

INGREDIENTS

- 2 eggs
- ¼ tsp salt
- ¼ tsp black pepper
- 1 tablespoon olive oil
- ¼ cup cheese
- ¼ tsp basil
- 1 tsp parsley

DIRECTIONS

1. In a bowl combine all ingredients together and mix well
2. In a skillet heat olive oil and pour the egg mixture
3. Cook for 1-2 minutes per side

4. When ready remove omelette from the skillet and serve

ONION OMELETTE

Serves: **1**

Prep Time: **5** Minutes

Cook Time: **10** Minutes

Total Time: **15** Minutes

INGREDIENTS

- 2 eggs
- ¼ tsp salt
- ¼ tsp black pepper
- 1 tablespoon olive oil
- ¼ cup cheese
- ¼ tsp basil
- 1 cup red onion

DIRECTIONS

1. In a bowl combine all ingredients together and mix well
2. In a skillet heat olive oil and pour the egg mixture
3. Cook for 1-2 minutes per side

4. When ready remove omelette from the skillet and serve

BEETROOT OMELETTE

Serves: **1**

Prep Time: **5** Minutes

Cook Time: **10** Minutes

Total Time: **15** Minutes

INGREDIENTS

- 2 eggs
- ¼ tsp salt
- ¼ tsp black pepper
- 1 tablespoon olive oil
- ¼ cup cheese
- ¼ tsp basil
- 1 cup mushrooms

DIRECTIONS

1. In a bowl combine all ingredients together and mix well
2. In a skillet heat olive oil and pour the egg mixture
3. Cook for 1-2 minutes per side

4. When ready remove omelette from the skillet and serve

BELL PEPPER OMELETTE

Serves: **1**
Prep Time: **5** Minutes

Cook Time: **10** Minutes

Total Time: **15** Minutes

INGREDIENTS

- 2 eggs
- ¼ tsp salt
- ¼ tsp black pepper
- 1 tablespoon olive oil
- ¼ cup cheese
- ¼ tsp basil
- 1 cup yellow bell pepper

DIRECTIONS

1. In a bowl combine all ingredients together and mix well
2. In a skillet heat olive oil and pour the egg mixture
3. Cook for 1-2 minutes per side

4. When ready remove omelette from the skillet and serve

CUCUMBER GUACAMOLE BITES

Serves: **4-6**

Prep Time: **5** Minutes

Cook Time: **10** Minutes

Total Time: **15** Minutes

INGREDIENTS

- 1 cucumber
- 1 cup Cilantro
- Chile powder

DIRECTIONS

1. Slice the cucumber into thick slices
2. Scoop out the center of the cucumber slice
3. Fill each cucumber slice with guacamole
4. Sprinkle with chile powder and serve

GREEK YOGURT AND TAHINI DIP

Serves: 1
Prep Time: 5 Minutes
Cook Time: 5 Minutes
Total Time: 10 Minutes

INGREDIENTS

- 1 cup Greek Yogurt
- ¼ cup green onion
- ¼ cup sour cream
- 1 tablespoon olive oil
- 1 tablespoon tahini paste
- 2-3 tomatoes
- 1 large cucumber

DIRECTIONS

1. In a bowl whisk together tahini paste, sour cream, olive oil and mix well
2. Add Greek yogurt, green onion and mix well
3. Serve with tomatoes or cucumbers

HAM AND DILL BITES

Serves: **4-6**
Prep Time: **5** Minutes
Cook Time: **5** Minutes
Total Time: **10** Minutes

INGREDIENTS

- 1 cup dill pickles
- 5-6 ham slices
- 1 cup cream cheese

DIRECTIONS

1. Cut dill pickles lengthwise
2. Spread cream cheese on every ham slice
3. Place a dill pickle on each ham slice and roll
4. Place toothpicks in each one and serve when ready

ROASTED ASPARAGUS IN HAM

Serves: 2
Prep Time: 5 Minutes
Cook Time: 10 Minutes
Total Time: 15 Minutes

INGREDIENTS

- 1 lb. asparagus spears
- 1 lb. ham

DIRECTIONS

1. Roll ham around each piece of asparagus
2. Lay asparagus on a baking sheet
3. Roast at 375 F for 10-12 minutes
4. When ready remove from the oven and serve

LUNCH

SPINACH FRITATTA

Serves: **2**
Prep Time: **10** Minutes
Cook Time: **20** Minutes
Total Time: **30** Minutes

INGREDIENTS

- ½ lb. spinach
- **1 tablespoon olive oil**
- ½ red onion
- **2 eggs**
- ¼ tsp salt
- **2 oz. cheddar cheese**
- 1 garlic clove
- ¼ tsp dill

DIRECTIONS

1. **In a bowl whisk eggs with salt and cheese**

2. In a frying pan heat olive oil and pour egg mixture
3. Add remaining ingredients and mix well
4. Serve when ready

TURNIP FRITATTA

Serves: 2
Prep Time: 10 Minutes
Cook Time: 20 Minutes
Total Time: 30 Minutes

INGREDIENTS

- ½ lb. spinach
- ¼ cup turnip
- ½ red onion
- 2 eggs
- ¼ tsp salt
- 2 oz. cheddar cheese
- 1 garlic clove
- ¼ tsp dill

DIRECTIONS

1. In a bowl whisk eggs with salt and cheese
2. In a frying pan heat olive oil and pour egg mixture

3. Add remaining ingredients and mix well
4. Serve when ready

SQUASH FRITATTA

Serves: **2**
Prep Time: **10** Minutes
Cook Time: **20** Minutes
Total Time: **30** Minutes

INGREDIENTS

- 1 cup squash
- 1 tablespoon olive oil
- ½ red onion
- 2 eggs
- ¼ tsp salt
- 2 oz. cheddar cheese
- 1 garlic clove
- ¼ tsp dill

DIRECTIONS

1. In a bowl whisk eggs with salt and cheese
2. In a frying pan heat olive oil and pour egg mixture

3. Add remaining ingredients and mix well
4. Serve when ready

HAM FRITATTA

Serves: **2**

Prep Time: **10** Minutes

Cook Time: **20** Minutes

Total Time: **30** Minutes

INGREDIENTS

- 8-10 slices ham
- 1 tablespoon olive oil
- ½ red onion
- 2 eggs
- ¼ tsp salt
- 2 oz. parmesan cheese
- 1 garlic clove
- ¼ tsp dill

DIRECTIONS

1. In a bowl whisk eggs with salt and parmesan cheese
2. In a frying pan heat olive oil and pour egg mixture

3. Add remaining ingredients and mix well
4. When prosciutto and eggs are cooked remove from heat and serve

ONION FRITATTA

Serves: **2**

Prep Time: **10** Minutes

Cook Time: **20** Minutes

Total Time: **30** Minutes

INGREDIENTS

- 1 tablespoon olive oil
- ½ red onion
- 2 eggs
- ¼ tsp salt
- 2 oz. cheddar cheese
- 1 garlic clove
- ¼ tsp dill

DIRECTIONS

1. In a bowl whisk eggs with salt and cheese
2. In a frying pan heat olive oil and pour egg mixture
3. Add remaining ingredients and mix well

4. Serve when ready

FRIED CHICKEN WITH ALMONDS

Serves: 2
Prep Time: 10 Minutes
Cook Time: 25 Minutes
Total Time: 35 Minutes

INGREDIENTS

- 1 cup bread crumbs
- ¼ cup parmesan cheese
- ¼ cup almonds
- 1 tsp salt
- 1 tablespoon parley leaves
- 1 clove garlic
- ½ cup olive oil
- 2 lb. chicken breast

DIRECTIONS

1. In a bowl combine parsley, almonds, garlic, parmesan, bread crumbs, salt and mix well
2. In a bowl add olive oil and dip chicken breast into olive oil

3. Place chicken into the breadcrumb mixture and toss to coat
4. Bake chicken at 375 F for 20-25 minutes
5. When ready remove chicken from the oven and serve

FILET MIGNON WITH TOMATO SAUCE

Serves: **4**
Prep Time: **10** Minutes
Cook Time: **30** Minutes
Total Time: **40** Minutes

INGREDIENTS

- 1 tsp soy sauce
- 1 tsp mustard
- 1 tsp parsley leaves
- 1 clove garlic
- 2-3 tomatoes
- 2 tsp olive oil
- 4-5 beef tenderloin steaks
- ½ tsp salt

DIRECTIONS

1. **In a bowl combine parsley, garlic, soy sauce, mustard and mix well**
2. **Stir in tomatoes slices and toss to coat**

3. In a skillet heat olive oil and place the steak
4. Cook until golden brown for 3-4 minutes
5. Transfer skillet to the oven and bake at 375 F for 8-10 minutes
6. When ready remove and serve with tomato sauce

ZUCCHINI NOODLES

Serves: 1
Prep Time: 5 Minutes
Cook Time: 15 Minutes
Total Time: 20 Minutes

INGREDIENTS

- 2 zucchinis
- 1 tablespoon olive oil
- 1 garlic clove
- ½ cup parmesan cheese
- 1 tsp salt

DIRECTIONS

1. Spiralize zucchini and set aside
2. In a skillet melt butter, add garlic and zucchini noodles
3. Toss to coat and cook for 5-6 minutes
4. When ready remove from the skillet and serve with parmesan cheese on top

GREEN BEANS WITH TOMATOES

Serves: **4**

Prep Time: **10** Minutes

Cook Time: **15** Minutes

Total Time: **25** Minutes

INGREDIENTS

- 1 cup water
- 1 lb. green beans
- 2 tomatoes
- 1 tsp olive oil
- 1 tsp Italian dressing
- salt

DIRECTIONS

1. In a pot bring water to a boil
2. Add green beans, tomatoes and boil for 10-12 minutes
3. Remove green beans and tomatoes to a bowl
4. Chop tomatoes, add Italian dressing, olive oil and serve

ROASTED CAULIFLOWER RICE

Serves: 2
Prep Time: 10 Minutes
Cook Time: 25 Minutes
Total Time: 35 Minutes

INGREDIENTS

- 3-4 cups frozen cauliflower rice
- 1 tablespoon olive oil
- 2 garlic cloves
- ½ cup parmesan cheese

DIRECTIONS

1. Place the cauliflower rice on a sheet pan
2. Sprinkle garlic and olive oil over the cauliflower rice and toss well
3. Spread cauliflower rice in a single layer in the pan
4. Roast cauliflower rice at 375 F for 20-25 minutes
5. When ready remove from the oven and serve with parmesan cheese on top

CAPRESE SALAD

Serves: 2
Prep Time: 5 Minutes
Cook Time: 5 Minutes
Total Time: 10 Minutes

INGREDIENTS

- 3 cups tomatoes
- 2 oz. mozzarella cheese
- 2 tablespoons basil
- 1 tablespoon olive oil

DIRECTIONS

1. In a bowl mix all ingredients and mix well
2. Serve with dressing

BUTTERNUT SQUASH SALAD

Serves: 2
Prep Time: 5 Minutes
Cook Time: 5 Minutes
Total Time: 10 Minutes

INGREDIENTS

- 3 cups butternut squash
- 1 cup cooked couscous
- 2 cups kale leaves
- 2 tablespoons cranberries
- 2 oz. goat cheese
- 1 cup salad dressing

DIRECTIONS

1. In a bowl mix all ingredients and mix well
2. Serve with dressing

TURKEY SALAD

Serves: 2
Prep Time: 5 Minutes
Cook Time: 5 Minutes
Total Time: 10 Minutes

INGREDIENTS

- 2 tablespoons lemon juice
- 2 tablespoons roasted garlic
- 2 tablespoons olive oil
- 1 tablespoon honey
- 2 cups cooked turkey breast
- 1 cup berries
- 1 cup green onions

DIRECTIONS

1. In a bowl mix all ingredients and mix well
2. Serve with dressing

SHRIMP SALAD

Serves: 2

Prep Time: 5 Minutes

Cook Time: 5 Minutes

Total Time: 10 Minutes

INGREDIENTS

- 1 tsp cumin
- 1 tablespoon chili powder
- 1 tablespoon lemon juice
- 1 tsp garlic powder
- 1 cup corn
- 1 can beans
- 4 cups romaine lettuce
- 1 cup salsa
- 1 cup salad dressing

DIRECTIONS

1. In a bowl mix all ingredients and mix well
2. Serve with dressing

CANTALOUPE SALAD

Serves: **2**

Prep Time: **5** Minutes

Cook Time: **5** Minutes

Total Time: **10** Minutes

INGREDIENTS

- 2 cups watermelon
- 1 cup cantaloupe
- 1 tablespoon honey
- 1 tablespoon mint
- 1 tsp basil leaves
- ½ cup feta cheese

DIRECTIONS

1. **In a bowl mix all ingredients and mix well**
2. **Serve with dressing**

CORN SALAD

Serves: 2
Prep Time: 5 Minutes
Cook Time: 5 Minutes
Total Time: 10 Minutes

INGREDIENTS

- 1 cup corn
- 1 cup cucumber
- 1 cup tomatoes
- ¼ cup avocado
- 1 tablespoon lime juice
- ½ cup Greek yogurt
- 1 cup salad dressing

DIRECTIONS

1. In a bowl mix all ingredients and mix well
2. Serve with dressing

SALMON EGG SALAD

Serves: 2
Prep Time: 5 Minutes
Cook Time: 5 Minutes
Total Time: 10 Minutes

INGREDIENTS

- 2 hard boiled eggs
- ¼ cup red onion
- 2 tablespoons capers
- 1 tablespoon lime juice
- 3 oz. smoked salmon
- 1 tablespoon olive oil

DIRECTIONS

1. In a bowl mix all ingredients and mix well
2. Serve with dressing

QUINOA SALAD

Serves: **2**
Prep Time: **5** Minutes
Cook Time: **5** Minutes
Total Time: **10** Minutes

INGREDIENTS

- 1 cup cooked quinoa
- 1 tablespoon olive oil
- 1 tablespoon mustard
- 2 tablespoons lemon juice
- 1 cucumber
- ½ red onion
- ½ cup almonds
- 1 tablespoon mint

DIRECTIONS

1. In a bowl mix all ingredients and mix well
2. Serve with dressing

GREEK SALAD

Serves: **2**
Prep Time: **5** Minutes
Cook Time: **5** Minutes
Total Time: **10** Minutes

INGREDIENTS

- 1 cup cucumber
- ¼ cup tomatoes
- ¼ cup red onion
- ¼ cup avocado
- ¼ cup feta cheese
- 1 tablespoon olives
- ¼ pecans
- 1 tablespoon vinegar
- 1 tsp olive oil

DIRECTIONS

1. In a bowl mix all ingredients and mix well
2. Serve with dressing

AVOCADO SALAD

Serves: 2
Prep Time: 5 Minutes
Cook Time: 5 Minutes
Total Time: 10 Minutes

INGREDIENTS

- 1 cup corn
- 1 cup tomatoes
- 1 cup cucumber
- ½ cup avocado
- ½ cup edamame
- 1 cup salad dressing

DIRECTIONS

1. In a bowl mix all ingredients and mix well
2. Serve with dressing

DINNER

SIMPLE PIZZA RECIPE

Serves: **6-8**
Prep Time: **10** Minutes
Cook Time: **15** Minutes
Total Time: **25** Minutes

INGREDIENTS

- 1 pizza crust
- ½ cup tomato sauce
- ¼ black pepper
- 1 cup pepperoni slices
- 1 cup mozzarella cheese
- 1 cup olives

DIRECTIONS

1. Spread tomato sauce on the pizza crust
2. Place all the toppings on the pizza crust
3. Bake the pizza at 425 F for 12-15 minutes

4. When ready remove pizza from the oven and serve

ZUCCHINI PIZZA

Serves: **6-8**
Prep Time: **10** Minutes
Cook Time: **15** Minutes
Total Time: **25** Minutes

INGREDIENTS

- 1 pizza crust
- ½ cup tomato sauce
- ¼ black pepper
- 1 cup zucchini slices
- 1 cup mozzarella cheese
- 1 cup olives

DIRECTIONS

1. Spread tomato sauce on the pizza crust
2. Place all the toppings on the pizza crust
3. Bake the pizza at 425 F for 12-15 minutes
4. When ready remove pizza from the oven and serve

CAULIFLOWER RECIPE

Serves: **6-8**

Prep Time: **10** Minutes

Cook Time: **15** Minutes

Total Time: **25** Minutes

INGREDIENTS

- 1 pizza crust
- ½ cup tomato sauce
- ¼ black pepper
- 1 cup cauliflower
- 1 cup mozzarella cheese
- 1 cup olives

DIRECTIONS

1. Spread tomato sauce on the pizza crust
2. Place all the toppings on the pizza crust
3. Bake the pizza at 425 F for 12-15 minutes
4. When ready remove pizza from the oven and serve

BROCCOLI RECIPE

Serves: **6-8**

Prep Time: **10** Minutes

Cook Time: **15** Minutes

Total Time: **25** Minutes

INGREDIENTS

- 1 pizza crust
- ½ cup tomato sauce
- ¼ black pepper
- 1 cup broccoli
- 1 cup mozzarella cheese
- 1 cup olives

DIRECTIONS

1. Spread tomato sauce on the pizza crust
2. Place all the toppings on the pizza crust
3. Bake the pizza at 425 F for 12-15 minutes
4. When ready remove pizza from the oven and serve

TOMATOES & HAM PIZZA

Serves: **6-8**

Prep Time: **10** Minutes

Cook Time: **15** Minutes

Total Time: **25** Minutes

INGREDIENTS

- 1 pizza crust
- ½ cup tomato sauce
- ¼ black pepper
- 1 cup pepperoni slices
- 1 cup tomatoes
- 6-8 ham slices
- 1 cup mozzarella cheese
- 1 cup olives

DIRECTIONS

1. Spread tomato sauce on the pizza crust
2. Place all the toppings on the pizza crust
3. Bake the pizza at 425 F for 12-15 minutes

4. When ready remove pizza from the oven and serve

ROASTED JALAPENO SOUP

Serves: **4**
Prep Time: **10** Minutes
Cook Time: **20** Minutes
Total Time: **30** Minutes

INGREDIENTS

- 1 tablespoon olive oil
- 1 tablespoon roasted jalapeno
- ¼ red onion
- ½ cup all-purpose flour
- ¼ tsp salt
- ¼ tsp pepper
- 1 can vegetable broth
- 1 cup heavy cream

DIRECTIONS

1. In a saucepan heat olive oil and sauté onion until tender
2. Add remaining ingredients to the saucepan and bring to a boil

3. When all the vegetables are tender transfer to a blender and blend until smooth
4. Pour soup into bowls, garnish with parsley and serve

PARSNIP SOUP

Serves: **4**

Prep Time: **10** Minutes

Cook Time: **20** Minutes

Total Time: **30** Minutes

INGREDIENTS

- 1 tablespoon olive oil
- 1 cup parsnip
- ¼ red onion
- ½ cup all-purpose flour
- ¼ tsp salt
- ¼ tsp pepper
- 1 can vegetable broth
- 1 cup heavy cream

DIRECTIONS

1. In a saucepan heat olive oil and sauté parsnip until tender
2. Add remaining ingredients to the saucepan and bring to a boil

3. When all the vegetables are tender transfer to a blender and blend until smooth
4. Pour soup into bowls, garnish with parsley and serve

SPINACH SOUP

Serves: **4**

Prep Time: **10** Minutes

Cook Time: **20** Minutes

Total Time: **30** Minutes

INGREDIENTS

- 1 tablespoon olive oil
- 1 lb. spinach
- ¼ red onion
- ½ cup all-purpose flour
- ¼ tsp salt
- ¼ tsp pepper
- 1 can vegetable broth
- 1 cup heavy cream

DIRECTIONS

1. In a saucepan heat olive oil and sauté spinach until tender
2. Add remaining ingredients to the saucepan and bring to a boil

3. When all the vegetables are tender transfer to a blender and blend until smooth
4. Pour soup into bowls, garnish with parsley and serve

CUCUMBER SOUP

Serves: **4**

Prep Time: **10** Minutes

Cook Time: **20** Minutes

Total Time: **30** Minutes

INGREDIENTS

- 1 tablespoon olive oil
- 1 lb. cucumber
- ¼ red onion
- ½ cup all-purpose flour
- ¼ tsp salt
- ¼ tsp pepper
- 1 can vegetable broth
- 1 cup heavy cream

DIRECTIONS

1. In a saucepan heat olive oil and sauté onion until tender
2. Add remaining ingredients to the saucepan and bring to a boil

3. When all the vegetables are tender transfer to a blender and blend until smooth
4. Pour soup into bowls, garnish with parsley and serve

SWEETCORN SOUP

Serves: **4**
Prep Time: **10** Minutes
Cook Time: **20** Minutes
Total Time: **30** Minutes

INGREDIENTS

- 1 tablespoon olive oil
- 1 lb. sweetcorn
- ¼ red onion
- ½ cup all-purpose flour
- ¼ tsp salt
- ¼ tsp pepper
- 1 can vegetable broth
- 1 cup heavy cream

DIRECTIONS

1. In a saucepan heat olive oil and sauté onion until tender
2. Add remaining ingredients to the saucepan and bring to a boil

3. When all the vegetables are tender transfer to a blender and blend until smooth
4. Pour soup into bowls, garnish with parsley and serve

SMOOTHIES

GREEN SMOOTHIE

Serves: **1**
Prep Time: **5** Minutes
Cook Time: **5** Minutes
Total Time: **10** Minutes

INGREDIENTS

- 1 banana
- 1 cup pineapple chunks
- 1 cup mango chunks
- 1 cup kale
- 1 cup ice
- ½ cup almond milk

DIRECTIONS

1. In a blender place all ingredients and blend until smooth
2. Pour smoothie in a glass and serve

WAKE UP SMOOTHIE

Serves: **1**

Prep Time: **5** Minutes

Cook Time: **5** Minutes

Total Time: **10** Minutes

INGREDIENTS

- 1 banana
- 1 cup coffee
- ¼ cup milk
- 1 pinch cinnamon
-

DIRECTIONS

1. In a blender place all ingredients and blend until smooth
2. Pour smoothie in a glass and serve

RASPBERRY SMOOTHIE

Serves: 1
Prep Time: 5 Minutes
Cook Time: 5 Minutes
Total Time: 10 Minutes

INGREDIENTS

- 1 cup raspberries
- ½ cup coconut milk
- 1 cup mango
- ¼ cup pear juice

DIRECTIONS

1. In a blender place all ingredients and blend until smooth
2. Pour smoothie in a glass and serve

CHOCOLATE SMOOTHIE

Serves: **1**

Prep Time: **5** Minutes

Cook Time: **5** Minutes

Total Time: **10** Minutes

INGREDIENTS

- 1 banana
- 1 tsp cocoa powder
- 1 cup almond milk
- 1 cup chocolate chips

DIRECTIONS

1. In a blender place all ingredients and blend until smooth
2. Pour smoothie in a glass and serve

PROTEIN SMOOTHIE

Serves: **1**
Prep Time: **5** Minutes
Cook Time: **5** Minutes
Total Time: **10** Minutes

INGREDIENTS

- ¼ avocado
- ¼ cup Greek Yogurt
- 1 tablespoon honey
- 1 cup low-fat milk
- 1 cup ice
- ¼ cup spinach

DIRECTIONS

1. In a blender place all ingredients and blend until smooth
2. Pour smoothie in a glass and serve

SUNSHINE SMOOTHIE

Serves: **1**

Prep Time: **5** Minutes

Cook Time: **5** Minutes

Total Time: **10** Minutes

INGREDIENTS

- 1 banana
- 1 cup almond milk
- Juice from 1 orange
- 1 tablespoon goji berries
- 1 cup ice

DIRECTIONS

1. In a blender place all ingredients and blend until smooth
2. Pour smoothie in a glass and serve

MANGO SMOOTHIE

Serves: *1*

Prep Time: *5* Minutes

Cook Time: *5* Minutes

Total Time: *10* Minutes

INGREDIENTS

- 1 cup mango
- 1 cup spinach
- ¼ avocado
- 1 cup milk
- 1 tsp vanilla extract

DIRECTIONS

1. In a blender place all ingredients and blend until smooth
2. Pour smoothie in a glass and serve

PEACH SMOOTHIE

Serves: **1**

Prep Time: **5** Minutes

Cook Time: **5** Minutes

Total Time: **10** Minutes

INGREDIENTS

- 1 cup almond milk
- 2 peaches
- 1 banana
- 1 cup ice
- 1 tablespoon honey
- 1 tsp almond extract

DIRECTIONS

1. **In a blender place all ingredients and blend until smooth**
2. **Pour smoothie in a glass and serve**

PUMPKIN SMOOTHIE

Serves: 1
Prep Time: 5 Minutes
Cook Time: 5 Minutes
Total Time: 10 Minutes

INGREDIENTS

- ¼ cup oats
- ½ cup puree
- 4 oz. Greek Yogurt
- 1 apple
- ½ cup almond milk
- 1 cup ice

DIRECTIONS

1. In a blender place all ingredients and blend until smooth
2. Pour smoothie in a glass and serve

THANK YOU FOR READING THIS BOOK!

Printed in Great Britain
by Amazon